Introduction

GU00838510

Most holidays or trips
However, if you, your
holiday or travelling a
enjoyment.

This guide contains h
issues. It explains how to travel comfortably and avoid travel sickness
or jet lag. There are also a large number of tips on how to prevent or
self treat common ailments experienced by travellers and holiday
makers.

The guide briefly outlines some of the common symptoms faced by
holiday makers and travellers. In addition the guide states when to
seek medical assistance for more serious health problems.

Here's hoping you don't need to use this guide on your travels but
just in case, don't leave home without it.

Enjoy your travels.

Contents

The Emergency Travel Kit

When abroad you will need medicines and dressings to help your self-care. Availability and quality of medicines and treatment may be variable overseas. If you have your own equipment you can be certain of its quality. Most medical equipment can be used only once.

Always have your own health travel kit. It may be the best investment you ever make. Take it on any trip abroad. You can purchase it from pharmacies, medical suppliers or some GP surgeries.

An Emergency Travel Kit is intended to be used during minor emergencies, but if properly stocked, can help you to deal with serious emergencies until professional medical help arrives.

Your Emergency Travel Kit should be passed to medically qualified staff as soon as possible. **You should not try to use syringes and needles yourself unless under medical supervision.**

ENSURE ALL CONTENTS REMAIN UNOPENED AND HAVE NOT PASSED THEIR EXPIRY DATE

For travel to more remote areas and depending on your own medical history, you should seek further medical advice prior to travel.

An Emergency Travel Kit will help you to cope with minor emergencies but it cannot substitute for the British Red Cross, St John Ambulance or other comprehensive First Aid training and certification, which we would recommend anyone to acquire as a useful skill.

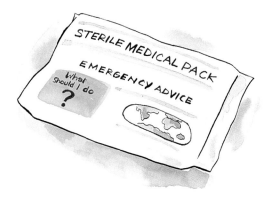

If you have children see the Child Care Section.

The Emergency Travel Kit (continued)

The kit should be large enough for you to clearly see and find anything you need quickly.

The location of the kit should always be kept in the same place so you can find it immediately. Ensure the kit is kept out of the reach of young children. Keep it apart from other medicines and supplies, and check it frequently to be sure to replace used and expired supplies.

The optimum contents of your kit should include:

Equipment
- Eye cup
- Fever strips (or thermometers)
- Safety pins
- Scissors
- Tweezers

Dressings
- Adhesive plasters, assorted sizes
- Plain gauze dressings (5 x 5cm and 10 x 10cm)
- Surgical tape (2.5cm x 2m)
- Adhesive tape and thin adhesive strips
- Crepe bandages x 2 (5cm x 1m)
- Gauze bandages: assorted rolled sizes

For treating cuts
- Skin sutures with needle
- Skin closures "butterfly"
- Alcohol swabs/disinfectant wipes

For injections
- 5ml Syringes x 2
- Needles x 5 – Gauges 19, 23, 25
- Cannulae x 2 – Gauge 23
- Alcohol swabs x 5

The Emergency Travel Kit (continued)

The kit should also include the following medicines.
Medications

- Antihistamine chlorpheniramine BP (piriton) or terfanidine (triludan)
- Antiseptic ointment – any brand
- Soluble Aspirin 300mg tablets (not for children under 13 years)
- Oily Calamine lotion
- Paracetamol (children's form if required)
- Sterile eye wash
- Toothache anaesthetic gel or Oil of Cloves
- Magnesium trisilicate or sodium bicarbonate tablets (antacid) or any other brand if you prefer
- Hydrocortisone 1% cream BP
- Clotrimazole 1% cream (antifungal)

Miscellaneous

- Plain soap
- Disposable gloves (or wash hands three times thoroughly and dry them between each wash).
- Tissues
- Add any special items, for example, an allergy kit, that may be needed by you or your family.

Useful items for emergencies

Try to keep the following useful items in mind, or keep a copy of this list with your Emergency Travel Kit:

- Blankets to keep the person warm.
- Sanitary towels can be used as a compress.
- Tea towels and linens for bandages.
- Magazines, newspapers, umbrella, cane, pillow, broomstick to use as splints.
- Small hand towels for padding a splint.
- Scarf, handkerchief or cloth table napkin to use as bandage or sling.
- Door or table leaf to use as a stretcher.

Travel Health Tips

Always carry any medications with you.

When travelling to another country
Try to find out how easy it is to use health care in that country. Establish the quality levels of treatment. Advice from your travel company or consulate can be helpful.

If you are leaving your children
Leave a consent-to-treat form with whoever is caring for your children.

Travelling across time zones
Jet lag (see Jet Lag section) can be reduced by timing the arrival at your destination to match your usual bedtime.

On arrival
Check you know the local emergency and medical service telephone numbers.

Certificates
Check with your travel agent before departure as to whether you need to take any vaccination certificates. Port authorities in certain countries require to see certificates as proof of vaccination.

Yellow Fever
The Yellow Fever certificate is the only one that has to be carried by international law. Many countries will want to see your Yellow Fever certificate if you have come from or travelled through (including plane touch downs) countries with Yellow Fever infected areas.

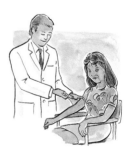

HIV Immune status
Port authorities in some countries require a certificate which shows your HIV immune status. The NHS does not provide this test but it can be performed for a fee by your GP privately or by a travel vaccination clinic. The result typically takes 10 working days to be available.

Childhood Vaccinations
These include polio, diphtheria, tetanus, pertussis (whooping cough), Hib, BCG (TB), measles, mumps and rubella. Certain countries sometimes require a confirmation from your doctor that standard vaccinations have been given to your child. Check with your travel agent, GP or travel vaccination clinic.

Travel Health Tips (continued)

When travelling with children

■ Make sure that the children know the name and telephone number of your hotel in case they get lost.

■ Give them enough money to make a phone call and make sure they know how to use the telephone.

When travelling to other countries

■ If you want to minimise the risk of diarrhoea do not drink tap water. (See Water Care section)

■ Bottled water may be safe, as long as it is factory bottled.

■ Traveller's diarrhoea can also result from drinks that contain ice.

■ Bottled carbonated drinks, beer and wine are usually safe.

■ Cooked foods are usually safe, but raw foods and salads (with lettuce or raw vegetables) can lead to abdominal/digestive problems.

■ Eat in restaurants that have a reputation for safe cooking. (See Food Care section)

Before Travelling

Arrange appropriate immunisation or check these immunisations are up-to-date. This should be performed at the time of booking or at least eight weeks before departure.

Notify your insurance company about previous/existing conditions eg diabetes.

Collect the following items together and ensure you know where they are in your luggage:

■ Non-prescription medications that you might need with you.

■ If concerned, take a signed repeat prescription with you, a computer print out or typed summary of your major health problems.

■ Passport.

■ Insurance papers and Form E111.

■ Emergency Travel Kit (See Emergency Travel Kit section or buy a ready packed one).

■ Sunscreen, hat and sunglasses.

■ The name and phone numbers of your pharmacist and doctor.

Food Care

Simple precautions can greatly reduce the risks from contaminated food. Remember you should **peel it, boil it or avoid it.**

- Always wash hands after going to the lavatory or before handling food and eating.
- Avoid food cooked in market stalls, however tasty it smells or looks.
- Avoid ice and ice cream in food.
- Avoid food that has been kept warm. Try to eat freshly cooked and piping hot food.
- Avoid food likely to have been exposed to flies.
- Avoid peeled fruit, salads, shellfish and raw food.
- Uncooked shellfish, such as oysters, are especially hazardous.
- Bread is SAFE, even if cut and left out.
- Avoid freshly squeezed fruit juice.
- Avoid sauces because they are often kept for long periods at room temperature and made from eggs or milk which are both ideal for bacteria to grow in.

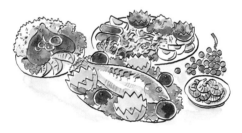

 This symbol denotes that you should follow guidelines on water care (found in the Water Care section)

This symbol denotes that you should follow guidelines on food care (found in the Food Care section)

Water Care

Diarrhoea, cholera, typhoid and hepatitis can all be caught through contaminated water. They can also be largely **avoided** by taking simple precautions.

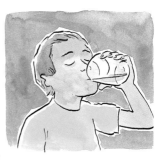

- If in doubt sterilise the water with disinfectant tablets.
- Only use bottled water, preferably carbonated, which has a tamper proof bottle top or comes in a sealed container.
- Avoid ice unless you are certain it is made from safe water.
- Avoid foods or drinks containing ice eg milk shakes, cocktails.
- In suspect areas use bottled water for cleaning teeth.
- Hot tea or coffee is usually safe, as is wine, beer, carbonated water, prepackaged or bottled fruit juices and soft drinks.
- Avoid or make sure you boil unpasteurised milk.

Take care in and around water

Water-based activities are often enjoyable but they can also be hazardous, especially for children. Fatal accidents or serious injuries often result from people being surprised by sudden changes in water conditions.

- Children should always be supervised by an adult who is a good swimmer.
- Never leave young children unattended by any stretch of water. This includes swimming pools and even paddling pools.
- Make sure water is deep enough for safe diving.
- Stay near the shore. Even the calmest of waters can be deceptive.
- If sailing, water-skiing, wind-surfing, jet-skiing, canoeing or some similar water-based activity, always wear a life jacket and make sure that adequate medical facilities are readily available.
- Do not swim after drinking alcohol or eating a meal.
- Remember to do some gentle muscle stretching or warming up exercises before swimming to avoid cramps.

Accidents and Simple Life-Saving First-Aid

WHEN SHOULD I GO TO ACCIDENT & EMERGENCY (CASUALTY)?

Most countries organise their health services in a very different way to those in the UK. Check with your local hotel, holiday representative or embassy for advice when you arrive (before any problems arise).

In countries that do not have a Family (Generalist) Doctor Service it is advisable to use the Hospital Emergency Room rather than decide for yourself which Specialist to see.

Go to Accident & Emergency (casualty)

If you believe that your problem cannot wait for a doctor's appointment or cannot be helped by self-care.

If you have time, phone a doctor first for advice.

Remember, most doctors have a system for seeing patients urgently during surgery hours. There may also be local weekend urgent problem surgeries or doctors who visit your hotel.

Go straight to Accident & Emergency (casualty)

If you have an injury that needs stitching, for example a bad or deep cut.

If you think you have broken anything.

Remember, **only call an ambulance if you cannot go or be taken to the hospital yourself**, or if you need a stretcher.

Be aware that in most countries there will be a charge for the use of the ambulance.

Accidents and Simple Life-Saving First-Aid

Do not use this method if you think that the unconscious person may have damage to the neck, back or any part of the spine.

First make sure that the unconscious person can breathe. Gently tilt the head back before placing the unconscious person into the 'recovery position' as shown in the pictures (**Steps 1 – 4**). Once in the 'recovery position':

■ Check that the unconscious person's hand is underneath the head, palm downwards.

■ Ensure the head is tilted back.

If you think the unconscious person may have a spinal injury, **only move them** if their head and neck are given extra support **and** if the head and trunk can be kept in line at all times.

Step 1

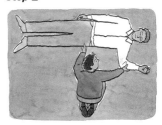

Step 2

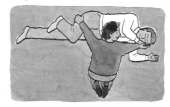

Step 3

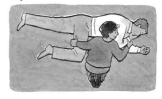

Step 4

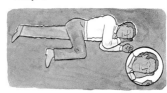

Note: *Remember to check the person's breathing and pulse at regular intervals.*

Blisters

Blisters occur when fluid collects under the top layer of skin. Blisters can vary in size from that of a pinhead to, in some cases, large swellings the size of a pencil end or bigger. Treatment is dependent on the cause of the blister. Causes include:

- **Friction** to any part of the skin leads to soreness, and in most cases, blisters. These usually occur on the feet as a result of ill fitting shoes or over walking, and on fingers and shoulders after carrying a heavy rucksack or suitcase. The blisters form quickly, are usually painful and contain a clear fluid.

- **Sunburn** (see Sunburn & Sunstroke section) is a common cause of blisters.

- **Coldsores** are due to a herpes virus which can be triggered in the skin around the mouth by strong sunlight and may sometimes form small blisters.

SELF-CARE:

What you can do yourself

Injury
If the blister is on the hands or feet, think of what you may have done that caused them. If it is the result of lots of walking or carrying heavy suitcases then stop this activity as soon as possible.

Clear blisters
- Blisters on the hands and feet can be very painful. This can be relieved by simple painkillers (such as Paracetamol or Aspirin) or putting an ice pack on the blister and surrounding area.

- Urea based skin creams can help soothe blisters.

- In cases where the blisters are very tense and painful, a sterile needle (or ordinary pin/needle sterilised by putting in a hot flame for five seconds and cooling) can be used to pierce the skin at the side of the blister once or twice, where it meets the skin. Clean tissue or gauze can be used to squeeze the fluid out. The area is best left open to the air. If there is a danger of contamination, it is advisable to keep the area covered.

Blisters (continued)

SELF-CARE:

Infection
White (pus-filled) blisters

- If the blister is very painful and painkillers have not helped and you cannot see a doctor within a few hours, piercing the blister will help (as discussed earlier). In this case, keep the blister covered.

Contact a doctor

- If the blister becomes full of yellow fluid or pus. Antibiotics and/or drainage under aseptic conditions are usual.
- If after piercing a blister, the skin becomes red, painful and tender.
- If blisters begin to increase in numbers and size. You may also notice that they become more itchy.
- If you have a pre-existing illness (such as diabetes) or are taking drugs, such as steroids which may effect your immune system.
- If you get more blisters with no obvious cause.

Contact a doctor immediately

- If you think that your blister(s) may be related to the medicine that you are taking.
- If you become feverish and generally unwell.
- If you think you may have blisters or shingles around the eye. The eye can become infected which may lead to scarring and blindness.

Broken Bones (Fractures)

A fractured or broken bone is an injury in which the bone tissue splits or cracks open and a space appears. This occurs if more pressure is put on a bone than it can stand. Sometimes the bone will appear deformed.

Sometimes the break causes a jagged end of bone to tear open the skin from the inside. This is called an 'open fracture'. This is serious as the bone can become infected.

SELF-CARE:

PREVENTION

Appropriate protective gear should be worn during sport or exercising. Care should be taken when skiing, cycling, motorcycling or taking part in water related activities:

- Helmets
- Elbow pads
- Knee pads
- Shin pads
- Life jackets
- Supervise children carefully. There is no substitute for adequate supervision, no matter how safe the environment or situation appears to be.
- Create a safe environment for young children.
- Teach safety. Help children learn how to protect themselves.

Is the bone broken?

It is sometimes hard to tell a dislocated bone from a broken bone. Both are emergency situations. The basic first aid steps are the same for both. (A dislocation occurs when a bone comes out of a joint).

Symptoms

- A visibly out of place or misshapen limb or joint
- Limited movement ability
- Swelling and intense pain
- Paleness
- No pulse is felt in affected limb

Broken Bones (Fractures) (continued)

SELF-CARE:

- Bruising
- Numbness and tingling
- Pain when putting weight on the limb

Children

Suspect a fracture or dislocation if a young child does the following:

- Does not start to use an injured arm or leg within three hours of an accident.
- Continues to cry when the injured area is touched.

Call immediately for emergency services/medical assistance if:

- The victim has a dislocation or broken bone, or if there is severe bleeding.

USEFUL FIRST AID TIPS

- DO NOT move the PERSON unless the injured area is completely immobilised.
- DO NOT move a person with an injured hip, pelvis, or upper leg unless it is absolutely necessary.
- DO NOT attempt to straighten a misshapen bone or joint or to change its position.
- DO NOT test a misshapen bone or joint for loss of function.
- **DO NOT give the victim anything by mouth as this will delay them having an operation, if they need one.**
- DO check the victim's airway, breathing and circulation. If necessary, begin rescue breathing, CPR or bleeding control.
- DO keep the victim still and provide reassurance.
- DO TRY AND PREVENT INFECTION. If the skin is broken by a fractured bone, or if you suspect there may be a broken bone under the skin do not breathe on the wound and do not wash or probe it. If possible, cover it with sterile dressings before immobilising the injury.
- DO apply ice packs to ease pain and swelling.

Broken Bones (Fractures) (continued)

SELF-CARE:

- Make an effort to prevent shock. Lay the victim flat, elevate the feet about 12 inches, and cover the victim with a coat or blanket. However, do not move the victim if a head, back, or leg injury is suspected.

- You may try to splint or sling the injury in the position in which you found it. Be sure to immobilise the area both above and below the injured joint and to check the circulation of the affected area after immobilising.

- DO seek help as quickly as possible.

Child Care

Children enjoy travel and on short trips there are usually few problems. There are a few tips to remember in relation to taking children abroad.

SELF-CARE:

Essential Points
- Arrange immunisations at least eight weeks before travel.
- Take any special medication or dietary requirements with you as they may not be found at your destination.
- Make sure that your children have identification on their person and details of their home address and place of residence abroad.
- Take some toys, games and refreshments for the journey itself or in case of delay.

With babies it is best to continue to breast feed if possible. Take proper precautions for sterilisation and preparation of feeds.

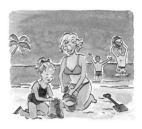

Infants and children are particularly susceptible to:

1. Dehydration
Ensure adequate fluid intake in hot climates.

2. Sunburn
Cover the children up, not forgetting protection for the head. Use lots of sunblock and search for shade.

3. Injuries and Accidents
Do not leave them unsupervised, particularly when swimming.

4. Diarrhoeal Illnesses
Follow advice on Food and Water Care. Beware of using local fresh milk or formulations using reconstituted powdered cow's milk as it can contain bacteria that can cause diarrhoea. Be aware that cow's milk is higher in salt and should not be used for rehydration. If there is no available refrigeration, **only use freshly prepared feeds** because bacteria are more likely to multiply if foods are not stored properly.

Child Care (continued)

Childhood Illnesses on Holiday

Your children are more likely than adults to have mild illnesses on holiday. Commonly these are diarrhoea, colds, coughs and sore throats. Treatment is to keep the child cool, comfortable and encourage them to take fluids.

You know your child best and if unsure seek a medical opinion.

Be on the lookout for serious warning signs, where medical opinion should be sought immediately. These are:

- If fever is very high and not responding to tepid sponging and Paracetamol.
- If your child is very weak.
- If your child is very drowsy or confused.
- If your child does not react when spoken to.
- If your child does not react to its surroundings.
- If your child has a headache and cannot sit up or bend the head forward.
- If your child has violet spots or rash which do not fade when pressed. (See Meningitis section)
- If your child is having breathing problems: gulping, gasping for air and is unable to speak or have a drink.
- If you think your child is in pain when breathing in.
- If your child passes blood in the motions or urine.
- If you think your child looks yellow (jaundiced). They may also pass darker coloured urine which appears the colour of a 'cola' soft drink.

This symbol denotes that you should follow guidelines on water care (found in the Water Care section)

This symbol denotes that you should follow guidelines on food care (found in the Food Care section)

Child Care (continued)

- If your child has persistent abdominal pain.
- If your child is passing urine more frequently with or without burning.
- If your child is not feeding for a good reason.

USEFUL ITEMS FOR YOUR MEDICAL CHEST TO TAKE ON HOLIDAY WITH CHILDREN

Treatment of Fever
Paracetamol/Calpol/Disprol

(60 – 120mg) up to four times daily – **Age:** 3 months to 2 years

(120 – 240mg) up to four times daily – **Age:** 2 to 6 years

(250 – 500mg) up to four times daily – **Age:** 6 to 12 years

Treatment of Diarrhoea
Oral rehydration solutions taken regularly (see Medicines section) will help replace important body fluids and salts. They are important whatever the age of the patient.

Treatment of Cuts and Abrasions
Cotton wool

Antiseptic solution

Plasters

Bandages

Treatment of Sunburn and Prickly Heat
Oily Calamine lotion

Chlorpheniramine (piriton)

Recommended Dosage of Chlorpheniramine:
(5 – 15mg) up to four times daily – **Age:** 1 to 5 years

(10 – 25mg) up to four times daily – **Age:** 6 to 12 years

Cystitis

The bladder lining can become inflamed and irritable due to infection. This leads to wanting to pass urine often, a burning sensation when doing so and in some cases bloody, cloudy or smelly urine. In more severe cases, the infection can spread to the kidneys and result in fever, pain in the back or lower abdomen, sickness or vomiting. Cystitis is more common in women.

Holiday (Honeymoon) Cystitis

Pain in passing water is a common short term problem during holidays for many women. The urethra can become sore and give symptoms similar to true cystitis. As a rule, antibiotics will not be required in these cases. Using a lubricating gel and changing your sexual position (to avoid friction at the urethral opening) are simple and effective ways of relieving 'holiday' cystitis.

SELF-CARE:

What you can do yourself

If you suffer cystitis frequently you could help prevent this by:

■ Drinking plenty of fluids.

■ Pass urine as soon as you feel the need.

Try to:

● Not to use soaps on 'sensitive areas'.

● Use sanitary towels only.

Sexually active women should minimise the risk of urine infections by:

■ Passing urine immediately after intercourse to help flush out any bacteria.

■ Using a lubricating gel to reduce friction during intercourse.

If you have cystitis

■ Fluids will help flush out the bacteria that cause infection and inflammation. Drink as much fluid as you can. As a guide, a glass of water (300ml) every 20 minutes is adequate.

■ A teaspoon of bicarbonate of soda in a glass of water every three hours will help relieve the burning sensation and pain.

Cystitis (continued)

SELF-CARE:

- Drink lemon barley squash.
- Cranberry juice is also helpful.
- Pass water as soon as you feel the need. Retaining urine leads to bacteria multiplying in the bladder.
- Try hydrotherapy. Shower the pelvic area for three minutes with warm water, followed by one minute of spraying with cold water.
- Hot water bottles can be used on the lower back or held between the legs or below the pubic bone to ease the pain.
- Simple painkillers such as Paracetamol or Aspirin will help.

When to seek the services of a pharmacist

- Potassium citrate mixtures will help to ease the burning sensation of cystitis.
- If symptoms of cystitis last longer than a day, a pharmacist may be able to dispense antibiotics (in some countries).

When to go to the doctor

- If the symptoms of cystitis are not improving within two days.
- If you have persistent blood in the urine with or without other symptoms.
- If you are pregnant and you suffer cystitis.
- If you have other illnesses which may be affected by cystitis or its treatment such as diabetes or a low immunity kidney problem.

When to seek medical attention immediately

- If you start to get increasing pain in the lower back.
- Have a high fever and are sweating.
- Also have sickness and vomiting

Diarrhoea (for Travellers)

Holiday makers and business travellers who travel to the USA, Northern Europe, Australia and New Zealand do not usually risk contracting travellers diarrhoea. The precautions and self-care strategies detailed are just like those you would follow at home. **In most cases, medical help will not be required if symptoms last less than five days.**

Most travellers suffer diarrhoea at some time during their stay in the Third World, Southern Sub Tropical Europe or Asia.

TRAVELLERS DIARRHOEA is a form of gastro-enteritis in people arriving in a new, usually hot country. It is caused by a type of *E. Coli* bacteria, common in that country, to which the traveller is not immune. Salmonella, amoeba/protozoa or viral infections also cause diarrhoea.

Babies and children

Children suffer travellers diarrhoea more often than adults. They do not have sufficient resistance (unless breast fed) and are more likely to forget or ignore basic hygiene precautions.

Baby diarrhoea is recognised by an increase in the number of motions that become more and more liquid. This can develop quickly and can lead to problems if left. A baby's diarrhoea often looks green.

Children are more susceptible to dehydration **particularly in hot countries.**

SELF-CARE:

What you can do yourself

PREVENTION

PEEL IT, BOIL IT OR AVOID IT

This is a maxim that should never be forgotten in high risk areas.

The bacteria is usually taken in from local food and water which has been contaminated by faeces.

TO REDUCE YOUR RISK OF SUFFERING DIARRHOEA

■ Observe the strictest personal hygiene. Wash hands before eating or drinking anything. Consider carrying baby wipes/alcohol wipes or cologne for this purpose.

Diarrhoea (for Travellers) (continued)

SELF-CARE:

- Eat only freshly cooked food that is still very hot, better still if it has been cooked in front of you.
- AVOID food cooked in market stalls – however tasty it smells or looks.
- AVOID sauces, especially those made from eggs or milk, as they are often kept for long periods at room temperature. Milk or eggs are ideal sources or environments for bacteria to grow.
- AVOID freshly squeezed fruit juice. Peeled fruit is SAFE.
- AVOID ice and unbottled water.
- Bottled water is ONLY SAFE if you see it opened in front of you.
- Alcohol is a disinfectant so it is usually SAFE. AVOID the ice!
- Bread is SAFE, even if cut and left out.

PREVENTATIVE TREATMENTS
Medicine to prevent diarrhoea is not recommended.

Antibiotics should never be used unless specifically prescribed by a doctor. The following groups of people are especially at risk:

- Women who are trying to get pregnant.
- Pregnant women.
- Women taking oral contraceptives unless condoms or another barrier method is used in addition.
- Children under 12 years of age.

If your trip is important for business or personal reasons and is of less than a week and you are prepared to risk/accept the possible side effects, there are a number of preventative medicines that you can obtain from a doctor on PRIVATE PRESCRIPTION before you travel.

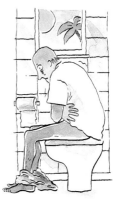

Diarrhoea (for Travellers) (continued)

SELF-CARE:

Preventative medication

- 60g BISMUTH SUBSALICYLATE daily.

OR 1 x 100mg capsule DOXYCYCLINE daily. (This medicine should never be used by children under 12 years of age, pregnant women or women trying to get pregnant.)

OR 1 x 200mg tablet TRIMETHOPRIM daily.

These treatments need to be started at least 48 hours before departure and continued for 48 hours after return.

If diarrhoea develops whilst away, DOUBLE DOSE for three days and also follow advice below.

If you suffer from a chronic medical condition or are taking regular medication please check with your own doctor on their suitability before starting medication.

TREATMENT OF DIARRHOEA
What you can do yourself

Nearly all symptoms will clear by themselves in two to five days, without any medicine.

Adults and children over 1 year

Avoid anti-diarrhoea medicines.

Only use anti-diarrhoea medicines if there is no fever or stomach cramps. If cramps occur stop the medicine.

There are two different and equally good approaches.

1 Starve for 24 hours or until diarrhoea slows, which ever is longer.

2 Eat only if hungry. Only eat plain bread, dry crackers, boiled rice, boiled potatoes or pasta.

For both approaches ensure that you

- Drink as much clear fluid as you can – if you have any ORS (oral rehydration sachets), use them. If not, use boiled water 250ml hourly interspersed with fizzy, sugary drinks and dry salty crackers. Add a pinch of salt to sugary drinks.

- Avoid caffeinated drinks, including colas as these stimulate the kidneys and cause further dehydration.

Diarrhoea (for Travellers) (continued)

- Avoid milk and all dairy products during the illness and for at least 72 hours following improvement.
- Once diarrhoea has stopped add plain foods such as bananas, vegetables or white meat the following day if you are feeling better.
- Avoid spicy or fatty foods, acid fruit and alcohol for 72 hours or until all symptoms have disappeared.

Remember: A woman's contraceptive pill will not give full protection when suffering diarrhoea. As well as taking the pill use other precautions during this time or for at least seven days.

Babies and children under 1 year

After each dirty nappy and as often as possible give your baby Oral Rehydration Solution (ORS) to drink. If the baby will not take ORS from a bottle then use a teaspoon and cup.

After the first four hours try and restart feeding.

Bottle Feeding

Give the baby ORS or a diluted soup of pureed pasta or potato. Avoid milk products for 24 hours. If weaned, give the child food as early as possible.

Breast Feeding

Increase the number of breast feeds. After each dirty nappy give your baby ORS to drink. If the baby will not take ORS from a bottle then use a teaspoon. Be sure you get extra fluids into the baby.

Avoid spreading infection

Wash your hands after you go to the toilet and after you change your baby's nappy. Clean the toilet often with disinfectant. Always clean under the toilet seat.

When to seek medical attention
If the child is under three months old seek medical advice early.

- If diarrhoea has failed to improve in three days.
- If you have an existing bowel disorder.
- If intermittent loose motions persist after your return.

Diarrhoea (for Travellers) (continued)

SELF-CARE:

When to seek medical attention immediately

- If diarrhoea is accompanied by high fever.
- If diarrhoea is so severe you cannot leave the toilet.
- If you have bloody diarrhoea.
- If you are also vomiting for longer than six hours.
- If you are becoming more seriously ill.
- If you are becoming confused or having hallucinations.
- If you are having increasing abdominal pain.

Contact a doctor

- If you are losing too much fluid (dehydration). Signs include dry skin, sunken eyes, dry tongue, drowsiness, less urine than normal.
- If you have a high temperature as well as diarrhoea.
- If you have been following this self-care advice and the diarrhoea goes on longer than a week.
- Your toddler has frequent episodes of diarrhoea.

Children over 1 year

- If symptoms go on longer than two days.

Babies under 3 months

- If diarrhoea persists for longer than eight hours.
- If the baby has a sunken spot on the top of its head.

Contact a doctor immediately

- If there is blood in the diarrhoea or the diarrhoea is red.

Babies and children under 1 year

- If your baby is drowsy or confused.
- If your baby does not want to drink for a few hours.
- If your baby is also being sick all the time.
- If your baby also has a high temperature.

Earache

Earache can be caused by eczema or wax in the ear canal. However it can also be caused by an infection in the middle ear. This is usually the result of a cold. The symptoms of middle ear infection are: earache, a feeling that there is a blockage in the ear, and a temperature. Sometimes fluid runs from the ear.

CHILDREN

When small children have a cold they often get a slight pressure in

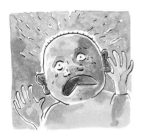 the ears. The lining of the air passages, which include the nose, throat, sinuses and middle ear can become inflamed as a result of infection. Mucus is produced and this can build up in the middle ear (the part behind the ear drum) if it cannot drain away into the back of the throat then earache is caused by mucus pressing on the ear drum.

After a few days, it is usual for swelling to go down and the trapped mucus drains. Sometimes bacteria grow in the mucus. The ear pain does not then disappear, and an unpleasant discharge can then be noticed coming from the ear. In some cases the infection only makes itself known by pus coming out of the ear. A yellowish damp patch will then be found on the pillow or in the ear.

SELF-CARE:

What you can do yourself

Laying the head a little higher in bed sometimes brings relief. You can use nose drops, decongestants, menthol sweets or steam inhalations, particularly before going to sleep. These are available without prescription from pharmacies. The pain may be relieved with a painkiller – such as Paracetamol.

CHILDREN

When children have a cold they are more likely to get middle ear infections. You may also give a painkiller such as children's Paracetamol. Make sure that at night the child's head lies higher than the rest of the body.

Earache (continued)

As a rule a middle ear infection without discharge does not need to be treated with antibiotics.

Contact a doctor

- If you have an earache with or without fever which does not disappear with a painkiller.
- If your ear starts to 'run' even if the pain has gone.

CHILDREN

- If, despite a maximum painkiller, the child still has a bad earache after 24 hours.
- If the child still has a slight earache after three days.
- If the child gets a runny ear.
- Have the child examined by a doctor if you suspect an ear infection, especially if the child is still too young to say so itself.
- When the area surrounding the ear is painful.

If following the earache you are concerned about the child's hearing, make an appointment with the doctor (on your return) to discuss whether a hearing test may be appropriate.

Contact a doctor immediately

CHILDREN

- If a child has a runny ear and the pain and/or fever does not lessen with treatment.
- If the child becomes drowsy.
- If the child is becoming more unwell despite the treatment.

Electrical Shocks & Injury

An electrical injury occurs when the skin or internal organs come in contact with an electrical current. The human body is a good conductor of electricity. Direct contact with electrical current can be potentially fatal.

While electrical burns can look minor, they can still cause serious internal damage, especially to the heart and brain.

Electric shock is a common occurrence for holiday makers because of trying to adapt electrical appliances to use local electricity supplies.

Causes:
- Young children biting or chewing on electrical cords or poking sharp objects into the electrical outlet.
- Accidental contact with exposed parts of electrical appliances or wiring.
- Lightning strikes.
- Flash of electric arcs from high-voltage power lines.
- Machines discharging electricity.

Most electric shocks are not usually fatal unless the person suffers from an existing heart or other medical condition.

The amount of damage depends on the site and extent of injury, the person's state of health, and the quality and speed of treatment.

Electric currents can cause injury in three ways:
- They can stop the heart. (Cardiac arrest due to electrical effect on the heart).
- Massive muscle destruction from current passing through the body.
- Thermal burns from direct contact with the electrical source.

The electric shock may
- Stop a person breathing.
- Break bones.
- Make a person deaf or blind.
- Cause paralysis.
- Make them wet or soil themselves (faecal or urinary incontinence).

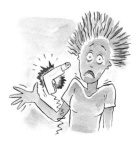

Electrical Shocks & Injury (continued)

PREVENTION
- RESPECT ELECTRICITY
- Use child safety plugs in all outlets.
- Keep electrical cords out of children's reach.
- Teach your children about the dangers of electricity.
- Avoid electrical hazards.
- Parents of small children should put safety guards on all electrical outlets and keep children away from electrical devices.
- Avoid using electrical appliances while showering or when wet.
- Never touch electrical appliances while touching taps or cold water pipes.

In an emergency
- DO NOT touch the victim with your bare hands while the person is still in contact with the source of electricity.

  If possible, shut off the electrical current.
- Remember simply turning off the appliance itself will not stop the flow of electricity.
- Unplug the cord, remove the fuse from the fuse box, or turn off the circuit breakers if possible.
- If the current cannot be turned off, use an object such as a broom, wooden or plastic chair, rug, or rubber doormat to push the victim away from the source of the current. Do not use a wet or metal object. If possible, stand on something dry and non-conducting, such as a mat or folded newspapers.

Once the person is free of the source of electricity
- Check the person's breathing and pulse. If either has stopped or seems dangerously slow or shallow, initiate first aid and resuscitation if appropriately trained.
- If the person has a burn, remove any clothing that comes off easily and rinse the burned area in cool running water until the pain subsides. Give first aid for burns.

Electrical Shocks & Injury (continued)

- If the person is faint or pale or shows other signs of shock put the person in the recovery position (see Accidents and Simple Life-saving First Aid section).
- Stay with the person until they receive medical help.

Electrical accidents often result in explosions which may lead to other injury. These may be obvious external injuries or concealed internal injuries.

Call immediately for emergency medical assistance if:

- The victim is unconscious.
- The victim has difficulty breathing.
- The victim has extensive burns.
- The victim develops significant delayed symptoms (see below).
- DO NOT remove dead skin or break blisters if the victim has acquired burns.
- DO NOT apply butter, ointments, medications, fluffy cotton dressings, or adhesive bandages to a burn.
- DO NOT touch the skin of someone who is being electrocuted.
- DO NOT get within 20 feet of someone who is being electrocuted by high-voltage electrical current until the power is turned off.
- DO NOT move a victim of electrical injury unless there is immediate danger.

Delayed Symptoms

For up to 72 hours after an electric shock the person may suffer the following symptoms:

- Fatigue
- Hearing impairment
- Panicky over-breathing (hyperventilation)
- Muscle spasm
- Difficulty in breathing
- Headache
- Chest pain (perhaps due to a heart attack)
- Loss of bladder or bowel control
- Muscular pain
- Loss of vision

If in doubt, contact a doctor for further advice.

Eye Irritation & Eye Infection

Eye strain/Tired eyes/Dry eyes

These are common problems on holiday and can cause a variety of different symptoms such as itching, burning, discomfort, heavy eyelids or short episodes of blurred vision. They can also cause headaches above the eyes. They are not painful and the whites of the eye do not go red, except in very severe cases.

These symptoms are caused by a drying of the skin covering the eyeball (conjuctiva). Usually the skin covering is kept clean and moist by blinking. Anything that over exposes the eye, reduces blinking or affects the tear gland secretions will cause sore eyes.

Long days, dirty, smoky or dry air and wind will all tend to overload the eyes own protective cleaning system.

Sore red eyes

Sore, red eyes are caused by the skin over the eye becoming irritated and red (inflamed). This is usually caused by one of three things;

1. An allergic reaction to something in the air (like pollen) or something liquid such as insecticide, soap or cream getting onto the eye and irritating it.

2. An infection, usually a virus or bacteria, but in the tropics fungal spores and some other rare infective agents can cause an infection.

3. Injury. Very commonly something gets into the eye and causes a very slight scratch on the skin of the eye. The body reacts as if it is a graze on any part of the skin. It increases the blood supply (making the eye red and swollen). The eye feels like there is still something in it even it may have been cleared away by blinking.

SELF-CARE:

What you can do yourself

Eye strain/Tired eyes/Dry eyes

- Rest/close your eyes for a few minutes.
- Rinse with cool, previously boiled water.
- If driving, use sunshades/sunglasses. Keep the windscreen clean, beware of open windows or open air vents blowing air directly into the eyes. Driving slowly can be very helpful.

Eye Irritation & Eye Infection (continued)

SELF-CARE:

■ Artificial tears/drops applied directly onto the eyes will moisten the skin and bring relief.

Allergy

■ Avoid the possible irritant.

■ Wear glasses to prevent any irritant blowing into the eye.

■ Rinse with cool, previously boiled water.

■ Try not to rub the eyes thereby causing further irritation.

■ Try sodium chloride (table salt) eyedrops to relieve the symptoms.

■ In some countries sodium chromoglycate eye drops can be purchased.

Infection

■ Wipe your eyes with cotton wool dipped in cool tea or previously boiled water. Apply the wool from the eye part nearest the nose and move outwards. Use the cotton wool once only and discard, repeating as necessary. This clears the discharge.

■ Viral infections are usually mild with little discharge and affect both eyes. Bacterial infections usually start in one eye and cause more discharge. Bacterial infections usually require antibiotic eye drops. Commonly, Chloramphenicol 0.5%, two drops in each eye every four to six hours will clear the infection. It is important that you continue the eyedrops for two days after the infection has appeared to clear.

Injury

■ If you suspect grit or dust has entered your eye and you can feel it on blinking, have a look in the mirror and if necessary turn the inside eyelids out. The grit or dust can be removed by rinsing the eye or using a piece of tissue. The eye should feel almost normal immediately.

Eye Irritation & Eye Infection (continued)

SELF-CARE:

When to seek medical opinion

- If you have followed all the advice and the symptoms are getting worse.

- If the eye becomes increasingly painful, red and sensitive to light.

- If after two days of artificial tears, eye drops or antibiotics, the symptoms have not cleared.

When to go straight to an eye specialist or casualty

- If you experience any loss of vision.

- If you cannot remove the "foreign" body such as dust, grit or insect.

- If you have any other medical condition which may slow down the process of healing/recovery.

- If the eye gets swollen, the skin around the eye becomes red, headaches increase and/or vomiting and fever develop.

- If you suspect that any object however small, such as a splinter of metal, glass, stone or spark from a fire or match has gone into or through the surface of the eye.

Fever

Fever is a raised body temperature of over 38.5°C (101°F). Your body temperature will be higher than normal and you will sweat.

Fever helps the body to fight the infection.

SELF-CARE:

What you can do yourself (aged over 12 years)

YOU MUST DRINK A LOT DURING A FEVER. You will lose more fluid. Make sure the ill person has enough safe water to drink.

Keep the room at a comfortable temperature.

Sponge the body with lukewarm water. This makes you feel more comfortable.

If you have a thermometer, use it. Place it under the armpit or in the mouth. If you do not have a thermometer use the backs of your knuckles and compare the temperature with your own forehead.

Aspirin is more effective in reducing a temperature than Paracetamol. (See the Medicines section for dosage guidelines). Do not give Aspirin to children under 13 years of age. Do not take Aspirin or Ibuprofen if you are allergic to them.

CHILDREN (12 years and below)

If your child has a fever then watch carefully for any further symptoms.

If your child is not at all its normal self, then give Paracetamol or Ibuprofen. Use twice the usually recommended children's dose if necessary for a maximum of 48 hours.

Contact a doctor

- If fever comes back after a few days of feeling normal.
- If fever does not go away within three days, and you do not know why you have the fever.
- If you feel listless.
- If you have been to the tropics or a very hot country recently.

Fever (continued)

SELF-CARE:

CHILDREN (12 years and below)

- If the child's fever returns after two days, and the child becomes unwell again.
- If the child is confused or drowsy, whatever its temperature.
- If the child is vomiting (being sick) all the time.
- If you think the child is in pain.
- If the child is short of breath.
- If the child has a fever and diarrhoea or vomiting or does not want to drink, after 24 hours.

Babies

- If the soft spot on top of your baby's head (fontanelle) is tight or bulging.
- If your baby moans when you lift its legs to change a dirty nappy.
- If the baby is being very sick (not just posseting).
- If your baby is not drinking much.
- If your baby gets diarrhoea.
- If your baby has a fit or convulsion.
- If your baby has a fever which does not go away after two days. Speak to a doctor about this, even if the baby seems to be normal and is drinking enough.

Contact a doctor immediately

- If you have a temperature of over 40°C (104°F).
- If you have a very stiff neck or vomiting. You may have a headache that does not go away as well and you may feel listless. (You have a stiff neck when you cannot bend the head forwards.)
- If adults have a rash.

Fever (continued)

CHILDREN (12 years and below)

- If your child feels very listless or appears to flop about, even if there is no fever or a low fever, your child could be very ill.

- If your child shows any signs of neck cramp or pain when bending the head, or vomits all the time.

Febrile convulsion

A fever that rises quickly may bring about a fever/temperature fit. This is called a febrile convulsion.

STAY WITH YOUR CHILD. Keep calm. The fit will usually only last for a few minutes.

Your child will not be able to talk and will have muscle spasms. Your child's eyes will be rolling.

After the fit your child will naturally go to sleep. Your child's breathing will be normal. (If your child is unconscious, breathing will be loud and very heavy.)

Gently place your child on its side or stomach, with the head down and to one side.

Contact a doctor for advice

Following a fit it is sometimes appropriate for your child to be admitted to hospital for observation and further treatment if necessary.

Hangover & Alcohol Intoxication

Alcohol has many 'side effects'. A hangover is a result of both the effects of alcohol and alcohol's waste products.

Alcohol causes excess loss of fluid. The dehydration that results causes headache, thirst, nausea, vomiting and tiredness.

In hot and humid conditions which cause dehydration, you are more likely to get a hangover. Salty and rich food also makes you more susceptible.

Most alcoholic drinks contain a mixture of two different alcohols - ethanol and methanol. Drinks high in methanol like brandy or rum produce worse hangovers. Gin and vodka based drinks have more ethanol and are less likely to cause hangovers.

SELF-CARE:

What you can do yourself?

PREVENTION
- Go easy. "Know" your limit. Most hangovers are caused by drinking more than your body can tolerate and allowing yourself to become dehydrated.
- Avoid drinks with a high methanol content.
- Try not to drink alcohol on an empty stomach. Try to eat some carbohydrate (bread, pasta, rice) before drinking. If you have not eaten and cannot eat anything drink a large glass of water (500ml) before your first drink.
- It is a good rule to drink at least $3/4$ pint (300ml) or a large tumbler of water with each or before each alcoholic drink. If you cannot face water, drink any dilute soft drink/juice that you can.
- Finally, before going to sleep, try and estimate how much you have drunk ($1/2$ pints or standard measure of alcohol) and ensure you have had at least an equal volume of water then drink one or two glasses of water extra before retiring to bed. Take a bottle of water to bed and if you wake early, still feeling dry, drink some more water.
- Before retiring take a high dose of Ibuprofen 400 or 600mg. (providing you do not suffer from indigestion or stomach ulcers.)

Hangover & Alcohol Intoxication (continued)

SELF-CARE:

■ Eat or drink something very high in sugar. The idea behind this is to help your liver burn/destroy the chemical, aldehyde, which is the first thing the liver breaks alcohol down into. It is the aldehyde that makes us feel terrible. High volumes of water will help the body to pass it out through the kidneys.

What you can do once you have a hangover?

■ Keep drinking fluid.

■ Eat high carbohydrate foods. Mix bread, potatoes, rice with sugar based foods to help the liver breakdown the aldehyde.

■ Provided your stomach is not sensitive take an "anti-inflammatory" drug like soluble Aspirin, Ibuprofen or related drug.

■ Paracetamol can help but is itself a little toxic in certain circumstances to the liver so is best avoided.

Headaches

Headaches vary greatly. Headaches vary in their site from a constant aching pain on either the scalp, cheeks, jaw, temple or back of the neck. Even on holiday, stress and tension are the commonest causes.

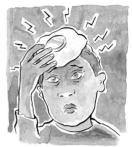

Dehydration is another common cause. This can occur after a long flight or journey. Consumption of alcohol or caffeine taken during travel can cause dehydration. Try to drink some water during the journey.

Other causes of headaches include heat exhaustion and hangovers and alcohol intoxication. Only very rarely are headaches more serious and most people would recognise the difference.

Migraine is caused by the blood flow changing to certain parts of the brain. A migraine usually affects one side of the head and blurs the vision/eyesight in one eye and makes you feel sick.

SELF-CARE:

What you can do yourself

- Ensure that you avoid possible causes of headaches whilst travelling. Drink plenty of fluid (non alcoholic). Other measures to avoid dehydration include keeping out of the sun and not drinking excessive alcohol.
- If you develop a headache
  1 Drink three or four glasses of water.
  2 Take Paracetamol (at least 1gram) or
  Aspirin (600 – 900mg) or Ibuprofen (200 – 400mg).

Do not give Aspirin to children under 13 years of age.

Headaches (continued)

SELF-CARE:

Contact a doctor

- If headaches occur with a fever, pain in cheek bones or bones over eyes (sinuses).
- If one sided.
- If a pattern develops.
- If occurring persistently on waking.
- If headaches persist for more than two weeks despite self-care.

Contact a doctor immediately

- If the headache is sudden, severe and unlike any you have had before.
- Associated with weakness, numbness, paralysis, confusion, odd behaviour, disturbed vision.
- Very sudden, explosive/"thunderclap" headache.
- If headaches follow a head injury/blow to the head.

Heartburn & Indigestion

Heartburn or indigestion is a burning sensation or discomfort. It is felt between the ribs and just below the breast bone. Sometimes a sour or bitter fluid comes up into the mouth or throat. Indigestion has many causes such as: overeating, obesity, irritant medicines such as Aspirin or Ibuprofen, alcohol, stomach ulcers or stomach infections. Sometimes the muscle valve at the top of the stomach does not work properly, often because the stomach has been pushed up through the gap in the diaphragm which the gullet passes through (known as a hiatus hernia).

The symptoms may worsen through anxiety, stress, smoking or alcohol, as these produce more and stronger stomach acid.

The symptoms may also worsen if you put on weight or become pregnant.

SELF-CARE:

What you can do yourself

Rest your stomach. Do not drink coffee or alcohol, and do not smoke. Avoid hot spicy food, such as curry.

Notice foods that bring on your heartburn.

Eat often and in small amounts. Take snacks like digestive biscuits and water. Chew your food well. Avoid any medicines which could irritate the stomach (most painkillers eg Aspirin and rheumatic pain remedies). Ask your pharmacist for advice or a suitable medicine.

- After your holiday has finished try to lose weight, even a few pounds.
- Take an over-the-counter preparation for heartburn.
- Avoid meals within two hours of bed time.
- Consider whether stress could be a cause.
- Go to bed on time.

Contact a doctor

- If you are getting stomach pains repeatedly, especially at night.
- If you are losing weight without trying.

Heartburn & Indigestion (continued)

SELF-CARE:

- If your appetite is reduced.
- If despite dietary efforts and antacids the problem lasts longer than two weeks.
- If you are over 55 years of age.

Contact a doctor immediately

- If you vomit and bring up blood.
- If your stools (bowel movements) look black.

Heat Exhaustion

In hot conditions we all sweat. If fluid loss becomes excessive we will become pale, feel weak and occasionally faint. This is called **heat exhaustion**.

The signs of this are:

- Weakness.
- Feeling faint.
- Pale colour to skin.
- The skin feels cool and moist.
- The pulse is weak and rapid.

SELF-CARE:

HEAT EXHAUSTION

What you can do yourself

- Lay the person in a cool place.
- Raise the feet.
- Encourage them to drink fluid (a litre of cool water to which one teaspoon of sugar and a pinch of salt has been added can be made up to help with rehydration).

HEAT STROKE

Heat stroke is not common but can be dangerous.

The signs of this are:
- The skin is very hot and dry. Not even the armpits are moist.
- The person has very high temperature 104°F (40°C).
- They often are, or rapidly become, unconscious.

What you can do yourself

- Cool the person as quickly a possible using the coldest water available.
- Call a doctor or take to hospital as soon as possible.
- Fanning the person will speed the cooling process which is vital in treatment.

Heat Exhaustion (continued)

HEAT CRAMPS

Sweating causes loss of salt and if excessive leads to cramp.

What you can do yourself

- Encourage plenty of SALTY WATER DRINKS.
- Repeat every hour until cramps go.
- Alternatively encourage eating salty snacks with water.
- Lay the person down and massage the affected muscles.

Hepatitis

Hepatitis is inflammation of the liver. When travelling abroad, there may be increased risk of exposure to the more common causes of the illness so prevention and self-care are important.

Causes and risk factors:

Hepatitis can be caused by bacterial or viral infections, infestation with parasites, chemicals (alcohol or drugs), toxins, or immune diseases. It can be short-term (acute), long-term (chronic), or life-threatening (fulminant). Hepatitis can cause permanent liver damage.

Some forms of infectious hepatitis are transmitted through blood products, some through eating contaminated food, some through sexual contact and some through unknown means.

Specific types of hepatitis include:
- Hepatitis A
- Hepatitis B
- Hepatitis C

Symptoms:
- Jaundice (Yellow skin and eye whites)
- Dark urine ('cola' coloured)
- Loss of appetite
- Fatigue/tiredness
- General discomfort or feeling ill
- Abdominal distention
- Generalised itching
- Loss of appetite
- Nausea and vomiting
- Low grade fever
- Pale or clay coloured stools
- Abnormal taste
- Abdominal pain
- Indigestion
- Nosebleeds
- Depression

SELF-CARE:

What you can do yourself
PREVENTION
Prevention of hepatitis varies with each type of infection. Some general precautions to reduce the chance of contracting hepatitis or other infections include:

1 Avoid contact with blood or blood products whenever possible.

2 Avoid sexual contact with a person infected with hepatitis, someone you suspect uses drugs, or a person with unknown health history. Practice safe sex.

3 Wash hands thoroughly after using toilet facilities or if there is contact with anyone's blood, faeces, or body fluids.

Hepatitis (continued)

SELF-CARE:

4 Hepatitis A and B vaccine is available if you are travelling to high risk areas (check with your local Travel Clinic).

Hepatitis A

In this case, there is an inflammation of the liver caused by the Hepatitis A virus.

The Hepatitis A virus is shed in the stools (faeces) of an infected person two to three weeks before symptoms occur and during the first week of the illness. Blood and secretions may also be infectious. This form of hepatitis is transmitted by eating or drinking contaminated food or water. The virus does not remain in the body after the infection has resolved, and there is no carrier state (a person who spreads the disease to others but does not become ill). The symptoms of Hepatitis A are similar to the flu, but the skin and the eyes may become yellow (jaundiced) because the liver is not able to filter bilirubin from the blood. Approximately 1 in 10,000 people suffer from Hepatitis A.

What you can do yourself

Prevention by following guidelines on water care is essential at all times. Transmission of the virus can be reduced by thorough hand washing after going to the toilet. This also applies if there is any contact with an affected person's blood, faeces, or any body fluids.

Rest is recommended during the first stages of the disease when the symptoms are most severe.

People with acute hepatitis should avoid alcohol and any substances that are toxic to the liver.

Contact a doctor

- If you have some or most of the symptoms listed above or are getting more unwell.
- If you think you may have been at risk.
- If you may be at increased risk of becoming more unwell through already suffering from another major illness.

Insect Bites or Stings

Most insect stings are themselves harmless. However, sometimes they may be serious. For example, if you are stung on the tongue or in the throat by a bee or wasp.

If you are allergic to bee or wasp stings it may trigger a severe allergic reaction. Reactions pointing to such an allergy are:

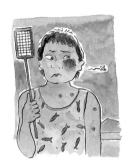

- Becoming generally unwell

- Swollen lips and eyes

- Generalised itching, possibly a rash

- Fainting

- Problems with breathing, such as wheezing and chest tightness.

SELF-CARE:

What you can do yourself

Most insect bites do not need any treatment. You can treat an irritating itch with do-it-yourself remedies or Hydrocortisone $1/2$% or 1% cream available from pharmacies. Ointments containing anti-histamines may cause an allergy and provoke itching and ideally these should not be used and are no longer recommended. Ask a pharmacist for advice.

Do-it-yourself remedies
Put some vinegar onto the spot where a wasp has stung. With a bee sting carefully remove the sting with a pair of tweezers without pressing on the venom sac.

If a tick will not come off remove it by smearing with some vaseline or butter. This blocks its breathing pores and forces it to let go, though it might take a few hours. Do not attempt to just pull it out, because you might break the tick's head from the body and it will be harder to remove the head from the skin.

Insect Bites or Stings (continued)

Contact a doctor

- If you can't remove the sting.

- If the bite becomes infected (bigger) and, despite antiseptic cream, the redness spreads.

- If you become unwell with a fever.

- In rural areas, if you have a tick bite which you can't remove, or redness develops in the area of the bite/sting.

Contact a doctor immediately

- With a bite on your tongue or in your throat.

- If you know you get dangerously ill from a bite.

- If you get blisters or a rash on another part of your body.

If stings trigger a severe allergic reaction these are the symptoms:

- Swollen lips and eyelids

- Increased generalised itchiness

- Difficulty in breathing

- Aches/pains, feeling unwell (wheezing)

- Becoming pale and fainting

If you have a severe allergic reaction phone for an ambulance.

Jet Lag & its Prevention

Travel to a different time zone usually disturbs the body's clock (the circadian rhythm) which regulates appetite, bowels, sleep and activity level and is controlled by a number of hormones and other chemicals. The readjustment takes place over a period of days. Readjustment takes longer if travelling in an easterly direction.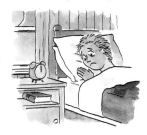

It can take up to seven days to re-adjust to a significantly different time zone.

SELF-CARE:

On long flights, the use of short acting sleeping tablets may help to shorten the period of jet lag. A short acting sleeping tablet can be taken to help fall asleep. If possible, ensure your sleep will not be disturbed for a few hours.

- For important meetings at your destination, always try to arrive at least 24 hours in advance of the meeting.

- Try to choose flights that arrive as close to night time as possible.

- Do not keep awake prior to a trip in order to make yourself tired. During the flight, drink plenty of liquids but avoid alcohol to prevent dehydration.

- Try to avoid caffeine as this can cause restlessness and disturb sleep.

- Avoid large meals.

- Avoid cigarette smoke.

- Avoid napping, which will delay your adjustment to the new time.

On arrival at your destination

- For short trips, maintain your old schedule of eating and sleeping at your usual time, if possible.

- Maintain a sensible bedtime schedule.

- If you usually exercise then do so at your destination.

Medicines

Remember good medicines can be expensive but expensive medicines are not always the best. It is also important to realise that in certain countries, such as France, it is common to supply some types of medicine in the form of suppositories where your British GP would give you tablets. Check with a local pharmacist as to how to take the medicine prescribed.

Names of medicines

The most common problem faced by travellers is varying brand names and even basic medicines do not share universal names in different countries.

Counterfeit medicines

Counterfeit medicines, creams and ointments are a growing problem world-wide. It is advisable to take any medicines you might need with you rather than hope to buy them from pharmacies abroad which may not be governed by strict laws relating to medicines. European community countries, USA, Canada, Australia and New Zealand all have good legislation with regard to medicines.

Dangerous reactions

Some medicines cannot be mixed. Certain combinations often cause unpleasant or dangerous reactions. So when abroad it is important to tell the doctor or pharmacist about the medicines you are already taking. For this reason ensure you write the names and dosage of your medication in a notebook or on a card that you keep with you at all times. If you receive medication while abroad try to make a note of what you were given. This will help your own doctor or pharmacist when you return home.

SELF-CARE:

Pre-existing Illness, Disease, Medical Problems

Ensure you take enough of your medicines with you. If you are away for longer than three months ensure adequate supplies are available at your destination. Take a list of medications with you. Use the proper (Generic) names – not brand names.

Medicine packaging and storage

■ Where possible use blister packs of tablets because they avoid being rattled around in your luggage and protect the tablets from crumbling.

Medicines (continued)

SELF-CARE:

- Tubes are best for carrying creams and ointments because they are less likely to allow dirt and bacteria to be introduced into the medicine.
- Pessaries and suppositories need to be sealed. In warm climates put them in the fridge to keep cool before use as they liquefy at 37°C (98°F).
- If travelling in a hot climate try to store the medicines in a dry, cool and dark place which is not accessible to children.

Allergic reactions

If you know you suffer from severe allergic reactions ensure you carry a card, dog-tags, Medalert bracelet or some other identification/medical condition item which explains what things you are allergic to. For example, antibiotics, peanuts, insect bites and such like.

If you are a person known to suffer from severe life threatening allergic reactions ensure that you have your adrenaline pen injector with you at all times when travelling. It is also advisable to travel with someone else who knows how to use the injector.

Antibiotics

These are commonly available to buy in many countries but you are strongly advised against buying them. If you think you require an antibiotic seek a health professional's advice at the earliest opportunity (unless you have a condition for which you have been regularly taking antibiotics in the UK and you are able to receive exactly the same medication and dose while abroad).

If you are allergic to antibiotics make sure the doctor or pharmacist you consult understands you have this allergy. Remember antibiotics are not effective against viral illnesses like colds and influenza.

Treatments you can make yourself

A number of useful medical products can be bought over the counter (OTC) but often highly effective treatments can be made by yourself from products available in the smallest general store. See the Emergency Travel Kit section for a list of useful medicines to have to hand when travelling.

Medicines (continued)

SELF-CARE:

Salt

Salt (sodium chloride) is probably one of the most useful chemicals to have with you when travelling. Use salt (half a teaspoon to a mug of lukewarm water) to make your own nose drops, mouthwash, gargle or eye drops.

Bicarbonate of soda or sodium bicarbonate

Bicarbonate of soda can be used for treating indigestion. Three teaspoons to half a mug of water (125ml). It can also be used in a dilute form (one teaspoonful to one mug of water (250ml)) to relieve the burning of urinary infections such as cystitis.

Calamine lotion

Use only OILY LOTION or OINTMENT because it can be rubbed in more effectively than the more usually available water based suspension. To convert a water based suspension to an oily one allow it to settle then pour off the water and add an equivalent volume of vegetable or mineral oil, such as olive or baby oil. Shake the suspension vigorously until mixed. Oily calamine lotion is a very effective anti-itch and cooling lotion. It is also useful to treat sunburn, insect bites, allergic rashes and any skin irritation. Hydrocortisone cream or other steroids are available over-the-counter in many countries.

Oral Rehydration preparations

With sugar and salt – Two level teaspoons of sugar and a pinch of salt to 250ml of boiled water. To this add 50ml of fruit juice, coconut milk or a quarter of a mashed over-ripe banana.

With powdered cereal or potatoes – Two heaped teaspoons of any of the following: wheat, maize flour, cooked mash potato, ground rice or pasta. This alternative is acceptable when baby milk must be avoided. Breast feeding should be increased, if possible, with additional rehydration solution used to supplement this if required.

Medicines (continued)

MEDICINES FOR PAIN

There are four levels of pain commonly experienced and these are the common painkiller alternatives to use if the pain continues.

All common self curing ailments are helped by third level pain killing strategies.

First level (low level pain)

■ Paracetamol - 500mg (known as Acetaminophen in some countries)

Adult dosage: Take two tablets every three or four hours, maximum dosage is eight Paracetamol tablets (4g) a day.

■ Soluble Aspirin – 300mg (not for children under 13 years)

Aspirin (acetylsalicylic acid) is the cheapest and most common painkiller available world-wide. Try to use soluble tablets and line your stomach with a little food.

Adult dosage: Take two or three tablets every three or four hours, maximum dosage is 12 Soluble Aspirin tablets (3.6g) a day.

Second level

■ Codeine – 15mg tablets

Adult dosage: Use Codeine with Paracetamol - one, two or even three tablets every four hours. Alternatively use a Paracetamol and Codeine combination available in many countries.

Third level

■ Ibuprofen – 200, 400, 600mg (also known as IBUFEN, NEUROFEN)

Adult dosage: Take 200mg or 400mg every eight hours. Can be taken with Paracetamol and Codeine.

Fourth level (high level pain)

Use a combination of eight Paracetamol a day as a base for adults:

Add up to three Codeine (45mg) four times a day and either three Soluble Aspirin or up to 600mg of Ibuprofen, four times a day.

If you are requiring a fourth line painkilling strategy to help your pain and you have not broken a bone, or know you are suffering from a serious illness then you must consult a Health Professional.

Meningitis

Meningitis is a rare illness caused by inflammation of the lining of the brain (meninges).

Meningitis is usually caused by infection. Virus infections are less severe. Bacterial infections, particularly meningococcal ones, can be fatal if not treated early. Meningococcal septicaemia (blood poisoning) can occur with meningitis or on its own.

The symptoms of meningitis may not all appear at the same time and can vary according to age. Symptoms associated with meningitis are:

- Headache (gradual onset, constant, increasing in severity and on bending the neck forward).
- Accompanied by fever, vomiting, drowsiness and sensitivity to light.
- A rash which forms and spreads quickly and looks like bruising.

The rash does not disappear when pressed against a clear glass tumbler but it is often harder to see in dark skinned people. Joint pains and fits may also occur.

For babies and small children, there may be fever, but with cold hands and feet, constant vomiting, fretfulness, a blank and staring expression, difficulty in waking, and refusing food. There can be a high pitched moaning cry and pale blotchy skin.

Early symptoms can be like severe flu and change with the passage of time. If you are concerned then phone your doctor for advice on the best course of action. If there is likely to be a delay then it is best to go straight to Accident & Emergency (Casualty).

If you have been in contact with someone who has had meningitis, you should contact their next of kin to find out any instructions from the hospital, or the director of public health, that they may have been given. Your GP can give appropriate advice after that.

Meningitis (continued)

Contact your doctor immediately

If the child continues to get more unwell and you notice one or more of the following danger signals:

Babies

- Difficult to wake.

- Vomiting (being sick) all the time.

- Fretful with high pitched crying.

- Refusing feeds.

- Appears pale or blotchy.

- If the soft spot on top of your baby's head is tight or bulging.

- Has a bruising-like rash that does not disappear with pressure from a clear glass tumbler.

- Fever (not always present).

Children and adults

Constant generalised headache with any of the following:

- Fever

- Vomiting

- Drowsiness or confusion.

- Sensitivity to light.

- Neck stiffness (it is painful and difficult to move your chin to your chest).

- The bruising-like rash that does not disappear with pressure from a clear glass tumbler.

Pregnancy

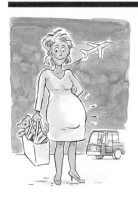

Make sure you have travel insurance that covers pregnancy

Travelling when pregnant is usually very safe.

Precautions that need to be taken are much the same as if you are not pregnant. However there are one or two important factors that need to be taken into account.

If you are unsure about how you are being treated then ask to be helped to contact your named consultant or midwife in the UK.

SELF-CARE:

What you can do yourself

- Most airlines do not allow travel if the woman is 34 weeks or more pregnant. Check with your airline before you go.

- Check the facilities at your destination in case of future emergency. If you are particularly at risk take advice from your midwife, obstetrician or GP prior to travel.

- Holiday immunisations need to be reviewed. Those involving live vaccines are best avoided. Consult your obstetrician or GP prior to travelling.

- It is useful but not essential to take any medical notes with you to your destination, together with a suitable translation of them.

- Do not miss any routine investigations, particularly in the first thirteen weeks of pregnancy.

- Anti-malarials are generally safe, but ask your pharmacist for advice.

- It is important when travelling to ensure adequate fluid intake and exercise.

Rabies

Rabies is a viral infection affecting the nervous system and salivary glands of warm-blooded animals, including humans.

Rabies is transmitted by the saliva of an infected animal that enters the body by a bite or open wound.

The virus travels from the wound along nerve pathways to the brain where it causes inflammation that results in the symptoms of the disease. The average incubation period is three to seven weeks but ranges from 10 days to seven years.

Areas affected

No reported cases have occurred in the UK since 1902 while Australia and New Zealand have been free from rabies for nearly as long.

Few cases have occurred in the last 10 years in northern Europe because of extensive animal-vaccination programmes including very successful oral vaccinations amongst wild carriers in northern Europe. The USA has seen an increase in cases in the last 10 years mainly in raccoons, skunks and bats.

The highest risk is to be found on the Indian, Asian and African continents.

Spread

Human cases usually result from a dog bite. However, rabies has been caused by the virus being carried by foxes, skunks, raccoons, bats and other animals.

SELF-CARE:

PREVENTION

AVOID THE BRITISH HABIT OF TOUCHING OR STROKING DOGS AND/OR WILD ANIMALS UNLESS YOU KNOW THEY HAVE BEEN VACCINATED. DO NOT ASSUME, ALWAYS ASK THE OWNER.

Rabies causes fear on the part of people who think they may have been exposed, but is now almost completely preventable and treatable.

Two types of treatment are available, they are:

■ Human Diploid Cell Rabies Vaccine (HDCV) which can be used as both a prevention and a cure. In its preventative role it acts like most other vaccinations to boost the body's own defences.

Rabies (continued)

- Rabies specific Human Immunoglobulin – this is an injection of antibodies which kills the virus. This treatment is only used after being bitten in high risk areas of the world.

When is the Preventative Rabies vaccine necessary?

The Preventative Rabies vaccine is only generally required if travelling to and planning to spend more than 30 days in high risk areas. These include Thailand, Pakistan, India, Nepal, the Philippines, Vietnam, Sri Lanka, Ecuador, Columbia, El Salvador, Peru, Guatemala, parts of Mexico and most South American, African and Asian countries.

Sex Related Diseases

Intimate sexual contact can lead to a number of symptoms and illnesses. Precautions to prevent illness are often forgotten or not used when travelling on holiday.

Sex related illnesses can cause discharge, itchiness, discomfort, lower abdominal pain and fever.

Women normally have a clear or white vaginal discharge. Infections can give an offensive smelling discharge, usually yellow with gonorrhoea and green with chlamydia which can cause irritation. With thrush, the discharge is non offensive smelling, white and "crumbly". This is not a serious illness and is related to changes in the acidity of the vagina, which can be taken advantage of by naturally occuring yeast.

Sexually transmitted diseases to be aware of are:

■ AIDS

People infected with the HIV virus will develop AIDS. This infects certain white cells and destroys them. It is transmitted in the same way as other sexually transmitted diseases and has no known cure.

■ Gonorrhoea

This more commonly gives symptoms in men in the form of a yellow discharge from the penis. Passing water is painful. Women often have no symptoms, however both partners need treatment.

■ Chlamydia

This gives an off-white discharge in men and pain on passing water. Women may have similar symptoms and vaginal irritation. Further treatment is required for both partners.

■ Trichomonas

This usually gives a profuse, vaginal discharge which is greenish, watery, smells offensive and causes irritation.

■ NSU

Non Specific Urethritis tends to give symptoms in men. Commonly, an off-white irritating discharge.

■ Herpes

Genital infection is caused by a different strain of herpes virus to that causing coldsores. In this case, there is tingling and burning before the painful blisters appear in the pelvic area and upper thighs. The groin can become swollen and tender when the lymph glands become inflamed.

Sex Related Diseases (continued)

■ **Genital Warts**

A certain strain of the wart virus can cause infection in the genital area and around the anus. Warts can form many months after exposure to risk.

■ **Pubic Lice**

Are transmitted by sexual or close bodily contact. Crabs appear as tiny white specks on the pubic hair. The eggs which are also white may also be seen.

SELF-CARE:

What you can do yourself

Prevention

There are only two ways to avoid sexually transmitted diseases. A stable relationship where both partners are aware of any health issues that may be harmful to the other and full disclosure occurs, or where no risks are taken and intercourse avoided.

Those in their teens and twenties are most at risk of trying new partners or sexual experiences whilst away.

It is important that you have protected sex at all times. Effective contraception and condoms will protect against unwanted pregnancy, infection and illness.

What is safe sex?

Sexual acts which involve no direct transmission of body fluid during the sexual act carry the least risk to both parties.

■ Avoid individuals at high risk such as prostitutes and drug users.

■ Avoid casual sexual encounters.

■ Be aware that asking a prospective individual whether they are "safe" is extremely unreliable.

■ Masturbation carries the least risk.

■ The proper use of condoms with other methods (such as spermicides and diaphragm) as necessary through all the stages of any casual sexual contact whether it be of oral, anal or vaginal type is always recommended.

Sex Related Diseases (continued)

If you have unprotected sexual intercourse, you will need post-coital contraception, commonly used is the "morning after pill". The "morning after pill" can be taken up to 72 hours after unprotected sex.

How to use condoms properly?

■ Products such as petroleum jelly (vaseline), baby oil and oil based vaginal and rectal preparations are likely to damage condoms and contraceptive diaphragms made from latex rubber. They may also render them less effective as a barrier method of contraception and as a protection from sexually transmitted diseases (including AIDS).

■ Latex condoms are best. Make sure they are not damaged or show signs of age. They should be kept out of direct sunlight.

■ They should be used before any sexual contact, whether oral, anal or vaginal in nature.

■ To prevent slippage after ejaculation, hold the base of the condom when withdrawing. This risk is minimised if the penis remains erect during withdrawal.

■ If the condom breaks, it should be immediately replaced.

Thrush

What you can do for yourself

If you have a white, crumbly discharge which causes irritation then you are likely to have thrush. Thrush can be helped by:

■ Wearing loose clothing, preferably cotton.

■ Using sanitary towels rather than tampons if the need arises.

■ Do not use soaps, disinfectants or bubble baths in the pelvic area.

■ A salty vaginal wash (made with one teaspoon of salt in one pint (600ml) of water) will cool the vagina.

■ Live natural yoghurt applied to the vulva with a sanitary towel or directly will help.

Sex Related Diseases (continued)

SELF-CARE:

- Antifungal cream (Clotrimazole) three times daily or pessaries (500mg), once only is sufficient.
- Some doctors recommend the male partner, particularly if uncircumcised should use the cream as well.

When to seek medical advice

- If symptoms of vaginal discharge and/or lower abdominal pain persist for more than 24 hours.
- If the male partner has symptoms of discharge/pain on passing water for more than 24 hours.
- If treatment for thrush is not helping after two days.
- If you think you may have genital herpes or warts.
- For the "morning after pill" if you have had unprotected sexual intercourse.
- It is best to have a check up from your local STD clinic on your return if you have been at risk whilst away.
- If your period is more than a week late.

If you are prescribed antibiotics

- Avoid alcohol as this increases nausea whilst taking the antibiotics.
- Take the full course of antibiotics.
- Ensure your partner is seen and if necessary completes any treatment.
- Do not have further sexual intercourse until clear of illness.
- Return to a clinic following the course of treatment to check you are clear.

Skin Rashes

Skin rashes are very common on holiday. They are usually a result of allergy (commonly to suncream), due to the sun itself (prickly heat), or infection.

Allergic rashes

Allergic reactions rarely occur the first time you use a new skin product. It often occurs on the second or third application. However, insect bites or "mite" infestation can lead to forms of allergic rash. This is usually very itchy. The most well known is scabies or head lice.

Tablets, taken whilst on holiday or even three weeks before the rash appears, can cause an itchy rash, with wheals (blotches) on the trunk or limbs. Antibiotics and "water" tablets are common causes.

Foods such as nuts, strawberries and shellfish may also cause allergic rashes.

Rashes due to infection

Rashes can be caused by bacterial, viral or fungal (yeast) infections. The rash often feels a little thickened, appears raised and may even crust. The most common rash is due to a fungal infection called ringworm. If it is crusty, it is likely to be due to impetigo or a similar skin condition caused by a skin bacteria.

Often, particularly in hot and humid conditions, skin infections develop and spread from cuts, grazes or insect bites.

Blisters can be caused by infection, commonly chicken pox, coldsores or shingles. (See section on Blisters)

SELF-CARE:

What you can do yourself

Allergic rashes

- ■ Stop using any suncream you may have used and think about any tablets or food that you may have eaten that could have caused the rash.

- ■ Cool the skin by applying ice or soothing lotion such as calamine. Oily calamine is better than the water based mixture.

- ■ $^1/2$% or 1% hydrocortisone cream or lotion spread very thinly is very effective.

Skin Rashes

- Anti-histamine tablets such as chlorpheniramine (Piriton) 4mg three times daily will help relieve the itchiness. Remember, it can cause drowsiness. It usually only has to be used for two to three days.

Rashes due to infection
- Try simple antiseptic lotions or ointments.
- Bathing with cool, salty, previously boiled water may help.

- If you have a bacterial rash which has not responded to antiseptics. A strong anti-bacterial ointment can be used. We suggest fucidin. This is often combined with hydrocortisone to combat the inflammation (dermatitis) in the skin.
- Allergic rashes can be treated with anti-histamines.

When to seek medical opinion
- If not helped by the above or if the rash/skin condition is worsening.
- If the rash is accompanied by a lot of pain.

When to contact a doctor immediately
- If the skin redness is spreading quickly.
- If red lines are tracking up from the infected area of skin.
- If the rash may be due to an important tablet that you are taking for an existing illness. It is important that this is confirmed as you will probably require new medication instead.

Go straight to Accident & Emergency (Casualty)
- Swelling around the eyes and mouth can be the first signs of a serious allergic reaction. You may also develop difficulty in breathing, wheeziness or feel faint and cold. **THIS IS A MEDICAL EMERGENCY AND IT MAY BE BEST TO CALL AN AMBULANCE OR TAKE THE PERSON STRAIGHT TO HOSPITAL TO PREVENT ANY DELAY IN GETTING MEDICAL ATTENTION.**

Sprains

Any sprain (such as a twisted ankle, shoulder or ankle) is caused by over-stretching ligaments and tissues of a joint. In serious cases the ligaments can partially tear or even tear completely.

SELF-CARE:

What you can do yourself

Directly after a sprain you can reduce bruising inside the joint by cooling it with very cold water, ice or a bag of frozen peas. For example, put a sprained joint into a bucket of ice cold water. The sooner this is done the better. It can reduce the time it takes for the sprain to get better. Do not strain or use the joint for three days. When sitting, keep the sprained joint high.

Ask a pharmacist for a suitable bandage.

Prevention

You can avoid sprains by staying fit. Always warm up before sport. Following a sprain it is important to train the muscles around the ligament properly.

Contact a doctor

- If there is no improvement after three or four days following the above advice.

Contact a doctor the same day

- If you are unable to stand on the foot.

- If you find the swelling disturbing and also if it occurred quickly, in just a few minutes.

- If you are in great pain.

Sunburn & Sunstroke

Direct sun can affect you in a number of ways. These changes can occur within a few hours from BURNING and SUNSTROKE.

The delayed action of the sun includes, ageing of the skin (small crusty spots, brown age spots, wrinkles) and SKIN CANCERS. Most of these effects only show themselves years later.

Sunlight can also have its benefits, including the making of natural Vitamin D, essential for strong bones, in addition it affects a part of the brain responsible for a good mood brain chemical (melatonin). Some conditions such as acne or psoriasis improve in the sun.

BURNING

The skin turns red and feels sore, is itchy and if severe it will blister and be extremely painful.

SUNSTROKE

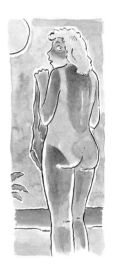

This is a type of radiation sickness, caused by ultra violet light. Symptoms are typically headache, dizziness, a raised temperature (fever), and vomiting.

PRICKLY HEAT

This is an allergic reaction in the skin often just to the sunlight alone, but increasingly it appears as a result of a combination/dual action of sunlight with either drugs or lotions, creams, perfumes, moisturisers or sunscreens.

Its symptoms are of a slight thickening of the skin, raised odd shaped wheals and itchiness.

PEOPLE AT HIGH RISK

- Children
- Pale skinned or very freckly individuals
- Naturally fair or red headed individuals
- People on certain types of medication (check the medication's information leaflet).
- Those taking trekking holidays involving long journeys in direct sun, especially through desert areas.

Sunburn & Sunstroke (continued)

SELF-CARE:

- Avoid direct sunlight. Stay out of the sun if your shadow is shorter than you are, (usually 10am to 2pm). Wear a wide brimmed hat or cap with a neck protector. Use a sunscreen or sun block.

- Avoid medications which increase sensitivity to sun or creams and lotions which may sensitise you.

- If trekking, cover completely with light cool long sleeved shirts and loose long trousers or skirts. If you do leave skin exposed, (remember your feet!), then cover it with a sun protection cream with at least a Sun Protection Factor of 20 or total sun block.

TANNING

- Build up your tan gradually.

- Limit yourself to a maximum 20 minutes (10 minutes in High Risk Groups), each side on the first day if sunbathing. This can be increased if you are using a new sunscreen by the sunscreen's SPF rating. For example 80 minutes if using a SPF 4 sunscreen.

- Never spend more than two hours on the beach at what ever time of day or 30 minutes when sun is high in the sky (and your shadow is shorter than you). Even if you do not burn you will run the risk of heat stroke.

SELF TREATMENT FOR SUNBURN & SUNSTROKE

SUNBURN

- Some find rubbing the skin gently with ice helpful, but do not over chill the skin.

- Cool the skin. Cool showers help.

- In mild cases apply an unperfumed "after sun" or simple moisturising cream.

- In cases of more severe soreness, it advisable to apply hydrocortisone cream (0.5% or 1%) available from pharmacies in most countries. A painkiller such as soluble Aspirin or Paracetamol may help.

- If itchiness is a problem, then an antihistamine/hayfever tablet will help.

Sunburn & Sunstroke (continued)

SELF-CARE:

SUNSTROKE
- Cool down by taking a lukewarm shower.
- Take Soluble Aspirin (Paracetamol for children under 13 years).
- Drink at least six glasses of water (2 – 3 litres) and continue frequent small drinks until you feel better.

When to consult a doctor
- If large areas of your skin have been burnt.
- If the burn has blistered.
- If babies have been sunburned.
- If toddlers have been burnt over an area of three times the size of one of their own hands.
- If you think the sun has reacted with a medication.

When to seek medical attention immediately
- If there is vomiting.
- If there are fevers, shivering, cold sweats, not helped by Aspirin.
- If you have palpitations or feel your heart racing.
- If the person is becoming increasingly unwell.

Tooth & Mouth Problems

Toothache

Toothache is generally the result of tooth decay which is often caused by poor dental hygiene, although the tendency to suffer tooth decay is partly inherited.

Pain from other locations can be felt in the teeth (health professionals call this referred pain or radiating pain).

Common causes:

- Earache.
- Injury to the jaw or mouth.
- A heart attack can also result in jaw pain, neck pain, or toothache.
- Sinusitis (inflamed air passages in the skull that surround the nose).

SELF-CARE:

Over the counter (OTC) pain medications may be used while waiting to see the dentist:

- PARACETAMOL 1gram every four to six hours (maximum 4g in 24 hours).
- SOLUBLE ASPIRIN 600 to 900mg every four hours (maximum 3600mg in 24 hours). Soluble Aspirin is not suitable for children under 13 years old.
- IBUPROFEN 200 to 600mg every four hours (maximum 2400mg in 24 hours).

Paracetamol may be used together with either Aspirin or Ibuprofen taken at the same time or separated by two hours so that breakthrough pain is covered.

FIXED READY- MADE COMBINATIONS ARE EXPENSIVE AND ALTHOUGH HEAVILY MARKETED ARE NOT RECOMMENDED AS THEY REDUCE YOUR CONTROL OF SELF MEDICATION

- Try a warm flannel or ice pack, either or both can help reduce pain.
- Oil of Cloves is an old fashioned "local" anaesthetic which numbs the tooth and is very effective.

TEETHING GELS or local anaesthetic GELS can also be bought for this purpose.

For toothaches caused by a tooth abscess the dentist may

Tooth & Mouth Problems (continued)

recommend antibiotic therapy and other treatments.

When travelling abroad we would advise that you politely decline any proper dentistry until you return to your own dentist (unless your absence is a long one). If in doubt phone your own dentist.

Call a dentist if:

- There is a persistent (longer than a day or two) or severe toothache.
- There is a fever, earache or pain upon opening the mouth wide.

Note: if the problem is caused by pain from another location of the body, you may need to contact a doctor.

Mouth ulcers

Mouth ulcers are white or pink sores found on the inside of the mouth or under the tongue. They are most commonly caused by a viral infection. They often recur at times of stress, other illness, or when we are run down. Very rarely they are due to a chronic bacterial infections associated with very poor dental hygiene.

SELF-CARE:

- Rinse mouth with home made saline solution (one teaspoon of salt in a glass of warm water).
- Apply local anaesthetic gel or other OTC preparation.
- Avoid food and drink that cause pain.
- Ensure teeth are properly cleaned (include flossing).

Contact a dentist

- If gums are bleeding.
- If you are suffering tooth pain.
- If sores do not get better within 14 days or recur frequently.

Contact a doctor

- If the problem occurs after a new medication.
- The cause of dental pain cannot be found.
- If the pain recurs very frequently.

Tooth & Mouth Problems (continued)

ACCIDENTAL TOOTH LOSS
Adults:
If a tooth is knocked out it may be possible for it to be re-implanted. It must be done within two hours, and if possible within half an hour.

Children:
First (baby) teeth usually are not re-implanted, a visit should be made on return home to the child's dentist to ensure no part of the root is left as this will distort the new tooth's growth.

- The tooth must be cleaned (milk is best).
- Transported either between the gum and the teeth of the patient's mouth or in a small container of milk (tap water kills the live tissues inside of the tooth).

Immediately contact a dentist
- If an adult loses a tooth and you can visit a dentist within two hours.

Contact a dentist as soon as practical
- For a check-up to ensure the tooth socket is clean.
- If a child needs dental attention.

If you are unable or too far from a dentist it is worth trying to put the tooth in yourself.

- If it is not very wobbly you may be successful.
- Try using chewing gum to hold it in place.

If you try this you must contact a dentist at the earliest opportunity even if it seems stable.

Bleeding gums
USUALLY CAUSED BY POOR CLEANING
Plaque builds up and causes the gums to become inflamed swell up and separate from the edge of the tooth. This allows more plaque and other mouth bacteria to get between teeth. This causes more inflammation and infection in the sockets as well as the gum.

Eventually the teeth loosen and fall out or the roots become infected.

Travel Sickness

There are some individuals who are particularly susceptible to motion sickness. The symptoms are those of nausea, lethargy, dry mouth, light headedness, drowsiness, headache and in some cases vomiting. The body over a matter of days can adjust itself to cope with motion sickness but thinking of your destination and holiday will be helpful in distracting your anxiety with the symptoms.

SELF-CARE:

What you can do yourself

Road
- Sit in the front seat.
- Slow the speed of the car particularly around corners.
- Ask the driver not to accelerate too quickly or brake too suddenly.
- Avoid reading material or viewing objects in the near distance whilst car is in motion.
- Look at the far horizon when the car is in motion.
- Avoid alcohol.
- Allow plenty of fresh air in the car to avoid a warm environment.

Sea
- Sit in the midship section. This is where the effects will be minimised of any sudden movements of the vessel in bad weather.
- If the symptoms of sea sickness are worsening, it is best to lie down, the relief is more profound if the eyes are closed.

Air
- Sit in the cabin section closest to the wings.
- Lie down and close your eyes or use a night shade.
- Avoid large meals and alcohol.

If these measures are not helpful or you are particularly susceptible to motion sickness then there are other ways to treat these symptoms.

Travel Sickness (continued)

SELF-CARE:

"Sea bands" are elasticated wrist bands which use a plastic button to apply pressure on the wrist at a point thought by acupuncturists to decrease the effects of travel sickness. It is particularly useful in children as it does not cause any side effects and is painless.

Certain drugs can be used to prevent motion sickness. Ideally, they need to be taken before travel for full effect. However, they can all cause a dry mouth, drowsiness and blurred vision and this needs to be borne in mind if driving or having to be at full mental power for subsequent meetings.

These drugs are available on prescription only.
Check their expiry date prior to planning to travel.

Commonly used Travel Sickness drugs include:

Hyoscine (0.3 – 0.6mg)
taken a minimum of half an hour before travel (lasts 4 hours)

Cyclizine (50mg)
taken a minimum of two hours before travel (lasts 12 hours)

Promethazine (25mg)
taken a minimum of two hours before travel (lasts 24 hours)

Cyclizine and Promethazine have the least side effects however their duration of action is longer so that you may need to be careful if you plan to drink alcohol on your arrival.

Alcohol will increase the potential side effects.

Vomiting

We vomit when the stomach will not tolerate the food it takes in. The quickest way for the stomach to get rid of the food is back upwards. This happens when the stomach is irritated by an infection or a poison/toxin. With an infection (gastroenteritis) there is usually diarrhoea and fever. When vomiting results from an infection, it generally lessens after 24 hours. A trace of blood may be seen in the

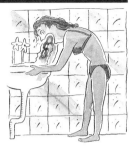

vomit. This is commonly from broken blood vessels in the gullet, due to retching and is no cause for concern. More blood than this could point to abdominal bleeding and you should call the doctor straight-away. Vomiting is common in early pregnancy.

CHILDREN OVER 1 YEAR

Children tend to vomit more readily than adults. The cause may be harmless but it can also be very serious. Usually the cause is physical, but vomiting may also be triggered by anxiety or fear.

SELF-CARE:

What you can do yourself

If you do not feel thirsty, it is best for the first couple of hours to allow the stomach to settle and do not eat or drink anything. Then begin with little sips of water or very dilute fruit juices or still lemonade. If this stays down, and you feel hungry, take some clear soup or water with sugar. Then switch slowly to more solid food like toast or plain boiled rice. Avoid milk and other dairy products as well as meat and fatty foods for 72 hours.

BABIES

At the start, try to give water, a teaspoonful at a time. If bottle feeding use $1/2$ oz water. If breast feeding, do not stop but give extra fluids. Avoid formula milk unless baby refuses all other fluid. In which case give it diluted, for example $1/4$ strength formula milk. When the vomiting has settled, change from water to $1/4$ strength powdered milk, and increase to $1/2$ then full strength if vomiting does not start again. If it re-starts, go back to the earlier strength that was tolerated.

Vomiting (continued)

SELF-CARE:

CHILDREN OVER 1 YEAR

Children can find vomiting frightening. So try to give reassurance by talking calmly when it happens. Try not to panic. Hold the child while he or she is vomiting.

Be sure to replace the loss of fluid and the salts and sugars it contains. Ideally do this with a fluid containing sugar and salt.

The best is a fluid called ORS (oral rehydration solution) which you prepare from powder or tablets available from a pharmacy. Ask a pharmacist for advice. Give small quantities of this fluid regularly.

Some children do not like ORS so it is best to give very dilute fruit juices or dilute still lemonade instead. A child that is vomiting and yet is drinking always retains a little of the fluid. If your child does not mind, try waiting two hours after vomiting has stopped and then continue with the fluids.

If the fluid stays down you can try some toast or crackers after a few hours. Do not force food on the child if it does not want it or if the child vomits again directly after eating.

If the child is vomiting yet has no other symptoms of illness and appears well otherwise, it may have eaten too many sweets or be upset about something. Vomiting accompanies most children's illnesses. Children with throat, ear or other infections often also have diarrhoea and fever. Usually this goes away within 24 hours. Children often vomit when they are starting a cold. Ask a pharmacist for advice.

BABIES

A mouthful of milk often comes up with a burp, 'posseting'. This is not serious. Coughing increases the pressure in the stomach. In babies and small children the muscle 'valve' at the entrance to the stomach then opens easily. However, if babies vomit forcefully (projectile vomiting) this could mean a blockage of the gastrointestinal tract (intestines). This usually only occurs in the first six weeks of life.

Vomiting (continued)

SELF-CARE:

Contact a doctor

- If you vomit for longer than a day and are not feeling better (even if you are aware of migraine).
- If you are pregnant and vomiting continuously for 24 hours.

Contact a doctor immediately

- If you are vomiting and have abdominal pain (stomach ache) that is getting worse.
- If you are vomiting blood or blood-like fluid. The fluid may look like "coffee grounds".
- With sudden headache and vomiting (not if you are aware of migraine).

CHILDREN

- If your child vomits for longer than one day.
- If your child also is not able to drink.
- If your child is generally unwell.
- If your child also has a high fever.

BABIES

At this age you should really always contact a doctor quickly when there is frequent vomiting.

- If for several hours the baby does not want to drink.
- If the baby also appears to have abdominal pain.
- If you find blood in the vomit.
- If the baby starts to vomit after a fall.
- If the baby is unusually drowsy and not reacting normally.
- If the eyes are sunken, the mouth dry and the baby appears to have lost weight.
- If the baby passes no urine or very little urine in 12 hours.
- If the baby continues to vomit forcefully (projectile vomits).
- If the baby has had no bowel movements for a whole day and its tummy feels hard.
- If you notice blood or blood staining in the motions.

Women's Health

Period Problems

Painful periods can ruin even the best planned holiday or business trip.

Painful periods can start soon after puberty. They may disappear after childbirth or develop after years of normal periods.

Sufferers get cramp-like pains in the lower abdomen at the start of a period. Sometimes they also feel faint or ill.

Symptoms most often pass after two or three days and rarely are they a sign of a more serious illness.

Periods are caused by either a narrow entrance to womb (cervix) or a slight hormone imbalance that causes a chemical (prostaglandin), to build up in the womb's (uterus) wall. This leads to spasm or contraction of the uterus.

Occasionally period pains in later life can be due to an infection of the lining of the womb or Fallopian tubes.

Even more rarely, period pains can be due to an over growth of the cells lining the womb spreading up the tubes and into the pelvis. This is called endometriosis.

SELF-CARE:

PREVENTION OF PERIOD PROBLEMS

■ Take plenty of exercise.

■ Eat a diet high in iron, calcium and the B vitamins.

TREATMENT OF PERIOD PROBLEMS

Rest and relax. Place a hot water bottle on lower abdomen. Alternating hot or cold packs may help. Try hot for two to three minutes, cold for 30 seconds, alternate them three or four times.

Camomile tea and a little root ginger can relieve the symptoms. Alternatively take either 3 x 300mg soluble Aspirin or 400mg Ibuprofen four times a day ideally beginning five days before the start and continuing during the course of the period.

Women's Health (continued)

Contact a doctor

- If it is not your usual time for a period.
- If your period is heavy and smelly.
- If your period is late and cramps are severe and painful.

Contact a doctor immediately

- If pain is so severe it hurts to move.
- If a period is late, the pain is severe and bleeding is unusually bright red.

BLEEDING BETWEEN PERIODS

Many women bleed between periods. It can be like a normal period or simple spotting. It does not necessarily mean that there is anything wrong.

It is common

- If in the first three months of a new pill.
- If an IUCD (coil) is present.

Use sanitary pads or tampons as normal.

Contact a doctor

- If bleeding is heavy (having to change super pad or tampon hourly for more than 24 hours).
- If more than 10 days in length.
- If bleeding occurs after sex.
- If you are over 35 years old.

Contact a doctor immediately

- If you also have unusual crampy pains, or a fever.

STOPPING PERIODS DURING YOUR HOLIDAY

Using any drug to stop your periods is not recommended. No preparation or drug, though safe and used very commonly world-wide is 'licensed' for stopping periods. If you wish to use them for your convenience it is therefore at your own risk.

Women's Health (continued)

IF YOU WISH TO avoid periods during your travels it is best achieved by continuing your oral contraceptive pill all through your visit.

Simply run two packets of pills together without a break.

If you are receiving Hormone Replacement Therapy (HRT) simply run two packets together, discarding the second pill that you take during the last two weeks of a packet. If using patches do not take the pill until you return.

Do not run more than three packets of oral contraceptive pill or 'HRT' together without a break.

If you are not on the 'Pill' or HRT you should consult a doctor at least six weeks before you travel overseas. This may allow you to start on a hormonal medication to prevent your periods.

We would recommend starting the 'Pill'. There are other hormones which can be used but they contain high dose Progesterone which can cause acne, headaches and are usually used for the treatment of very heavy periods. Their use, though safe, has not been fully evaluated for this purpose.

Wounds

The aim of treating wounds is to stop any bleeding, prevent infection and to encourage healing as fast as possible with the least possible after-effects.

SELF-CARE:

What you can do yourself

Minor surface wounds

When you have a wound be sure to clean it carefully. Rinse away sand and other dirt under flowing water. Ask your pharmacist for a suitable disinfectant and advice about dressing the wound correctly. Cover minor surface wounds with fabric plasters. Change the plasters every two days. Change more often if blood is coming through the plaster or it gets wet. If the wound is bleeding try to stop it by pressing down on the wound (remember to wash your hands first). Bleeding from a wound on the arm or leg can be helped by lifting the limb higher than the body.

Contact a doctor

- If you get a fever.

- If the wound starts to hurt again after a few days.

- If the wound is not healing.

- If you have never had a tetanus vaccination or your vaccination was over ten years ago.

Contact a doctor immediately

- If the bleeding is serious.

- If it is not possible to clean a wound properly.

- If an open wound goes deeper than $1/10$ inch (2mm). It must be stitched within eight hours.

- If it is due to a human or animal bite.

- If the red area around the wound becomes larger than $1/4$ inch (5mm), possibly with red lines going down the arms or legs. This can point to an infection. A fever may then also occur.

Travel Health Insurance

- **DON'T, DON'T, DON'T GO ABROAD WITHOUT TRAVEL HEALTH INSURANCE**
- Make travel health insurance arrangements as soon as you confirm your holiday and do not leave it too late.
- If you possess private travel health insurance for use in this country, it may cover you abroad. (If you travel frequently to foreign destinations then it will be helpful if this is covered in your policy.)
- Tailor your holiday/travel health insurance according to your individual requirements.
- Take details of your travel insurance with you.
- Take your NHS Card with you. If you do not have it, you will need to phone your local health authority and ask for the registration department they will issue a new one.

IF YOU BECOME ILL ABROAD WHO CAN HELP?

- Travel representative
- Hotel management
- A local state hospital, otherwise private care if available
- The British Consulate in that country
- Your health insurance company will provide you with details of who to contact locally, or back at home, in case of difficulty.

REMEMBER TO

- Advise medical personnel of your past medical history, medication you may be taking and any allergies.
- Keep invoices for all investigations and treatment including drugs.
- If appropriate, claim re-imbursement prior to leaving.

Treatment when abroad

- Ensure you follow the strict guidelines of your insurance policy.
- It is advisable to make any claim as soon as possible.
- It is advisable if claiming treatment on the Form E111, (see Form E111 section) to put in your claim immediately on return home.

Form E111

The European Economic Area (EEA) consists of the member states of the European Community plus Iceland, Liechtenstein and Norway. If you or any of your dependents are suddenly taken ill or have an accident during a visit to any of these countries, free or reduced-cost emergency treatment is available, in most cases on production of a valid Form E111. Only state provided emergency treatment is covered. You will receive treatment on the same terms as nationals of the country. Private treatment is generally not covered. Each of the EEA countries has its own rules for state medical provision.

Who is eligible for an E111?

You are eligible to obtain Form E111 if you are resident in the UK and you are:

- A UK national
- A national of any other EEA country
- A refugee or stateless individual
- A widow receiving a UK state pension or Widows Benefit whose late husband was a national of a EEA country, living in the UK at the time of his death

E111 ceases to be valid once you live outside the UK.

If you have dual British/foreign nationality or if you do not have a British passport but you consider you are a British citizen for the purposes of E111, you must provide evidence of your British nationality. Enquiries should be addressed to:

Home Office
Immigration & Nationality Departments
India Buildings (3rd Floor)
Water Street
Liverpool L2 0QN

If you are a EEA national, a stateless person or a refugee working in the UK, but paying social security contributions to EEA country, you should obtain your E111 from the institution to which you pay your contributions.

Obtaining Form E111

The form can be obtained from main post offices. On completion of the application, it needs to be returned, where the E111 will be stamped and signed and returned to you. Keep it safe, preferably with your passport, and carry it with you when travelling within the EEA.

Form E111 (continued)

Your E111 remains valid indefinitely so long as you remain ordinarily resident in the UK. You will only need to apply for another E111 if you use it to claim for treatment or if you mislay it.

Form E111 covers both you, your spouse and your dependent children up to the age of 16, or 19 if they are still in full time education. You should apply for an amended E111 when your children pass those ages.

If you change address you should amend Section 1 of your E111.

It is sensible to keep a photocopy of your E111 with the original. In any case, a photocopy is required, and retained when you apply for treatment in Belgium, France, Germany, Italy, the Netherlands and Spain.

Points to Consider on Returning Home

Most travellers return feeling well from their holidays or business trips. However, it is important that a number of precautions are taken once you return home safely:

- Check with the airline or customs that medication prescribed abroad is legal in the UK.
- Continue anti-malarial tablets for one month after your return.
- With malaria, symptoms can occur up to nine months following your return.
- Continue any medication that you were prescribed when abroad.
- It is best to inform your doctor at the time of consultation where you have been travelling abroad.
- Ensure details of your treatment whilst abroad are given to your surgery.
- Inform the blood transfusion service before donating blood if you have been unwell when abroad.

Contact your Health Centre (GP or Practice Nurse), or Occupational Health Service if:

- You become unwell following your return
- You are concerned that you are a Health Risk, particularly as a result of sexually transmitted diseases or insect or animal bites.
- You suffered diarrhoea whilst on holiday or shortly after your return and it is **persistent**.
- You have had, or suspect, food poisoning and your job involves handling food, it is best to inform your employer (or your occupational health department).

Remember if you were unwell when abroad and are still ill on your return, or in some cases become unwell sometime after your return, then ensure that:

- You inform the airline or other transport organisations of your illness.
- In cases of serious illness, your doctor will then be able to liaise with the appropriate authorities.

If unsure, seek medical advice at point of arrival.

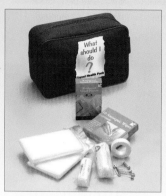

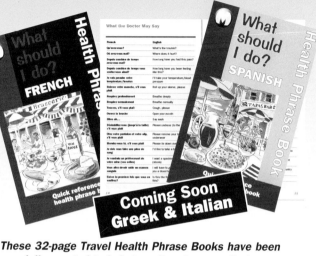

Quick reference health care guide

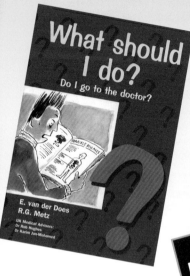

This easy to use, step-by-step guide details more than 50 minor illnesses.

Ideal as a home reference for common family ailments.

Provides specific health information to care for babies and children.

Written by leading GPs and used by 3million people in the UK.

Keep it by your phone